The Snacks and Appetizers Cookbook for the Anti-Inflammatory Diet

Mouthwatering Anti-Inflammatory Recipes To Fight Inflammation on Breaks

By
Olga Jones

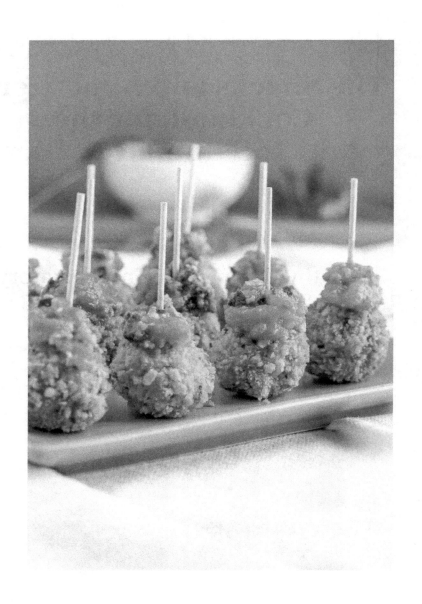

additional rights reserved.

The information in the following pages is broadly considered a truthful and accurate account of facts and as such, any inattention, use, or misuse of the information in question by the reader will render any resulting actions solely under their purview. There are no scenarios in which the publisher or the original author of this work can be in any fashion deemed liable for any hardship or damages that may befall them after undertaking information described herein.

Additionally, the information in the following pages is intended only for informational purposes and should thus be thought of as universal. As befitting its nature, it is presented without assurance regarding its prolonged validity or interim quality. Trademarks that are mentioned are done without written consent and can in no way be considered an endorsement from the trademark holder.

Table of Contents

INTRODUCTION

What is the Anti-Inflammatory Diet?

The anti-inflammatory diet is the best choice for your health if you have conditions that cause inflammation. Such conditions are asthma, chronic peptic ulcer, tuberculosis, rheumatoid arthritis, periodontitis, Crohn's disease, sinusitis, active hepatitis, etc. Along with medical treatment, proper nutrition is very important. An anti-inflammatory diet can help to reduce the pain from inflammation for a few notches. Such a diet isn't a panacea but a significant help in any treatment. Inflammation is a natural response of your body to infections, injuries, and illnesses. The classic symptoms of inflammation are redness, pain, heat, and swelling. Nevertheless, some diseases don't have any symptoms. Such illnesses are diabetes, heart disease, cancer, etc. That's why we should care about our health permanently and an anti-inflammatory diet is one of the ways for it.

Inflammation is your immune system's response to injury or unwanted microbes in your body. It is a natural process and vital part of your body's healing process.

When inflammation becomes systemic and chronic, however, it becomes a problem, and measures need to be taken. This type of inflammation serves no purpose, and can cause a lot of harm to the body.

This book has a LOT of recipes, and not every recipe might work for you. For example, if you're allergic to dairy or gluten, the recipes containing those ingredients will cause more harm than good. However, substitutions are possible for all of these, so you will be fine following this book as long as you keep an eye on the ingredients and use a bit of creativity where you have to! Once you understand the fundamentals of the diet, you will be fully equipped to create your own recipes from scratch!This is the most important information that you should know before starting a diet. Any diet is not a magic remedy for all diseases; it is a support for the body during a difficult time of treatment. Start your new healthy life from one small step and you will see the huge results within half a year. You can be sure that your body will be thankful to you by giving you a fresh look and energy for new achievements.

SIDES

Beet Hummus

Time To Prepare: five minutes

Time to Cook: 0 minutes

Yield: Servings 2

Ingredients:
- ¼ tsp of chili flakes
- ½ cup of olive oil
- ½ tsp of oregano
- ½ tsp of salt
- 1 ½ tsp of cumin
- 1 ¾ cup of chickpeas
- 1 clove of garlic
- 1 nub of fresh ginger
- 1 skinless roasted beet
- 1 tsp of curry
- 1 tsp of maple syrup
- 2 tbsp. of sunflower seeds
- Juice of one lemon

Directions:

Blend all together the ingredients in a food processor until they're smooth and decorate them with sunflower seeds. Enjoy!

Caramelized Pears and Onions

Time To Prepare: five minutes

Time to Cook: thirty-five minutes

Yield: Servings 4

Ingredients:
- 1 tablespoon olive oil

- 2 firm red pears, cored and quartered

- 2 red onion, cut into wedges

- Salt and pepper, to taste

Directions:
1. Preheat the oven to 425 degrees F

2. Put the pears and onion on a baking tray

3. Sprinkle with olive oil

4. Sprinkle with salt and pepper

5. Bake using your oven for a little more than half an hour

6. Serve and enjoy!

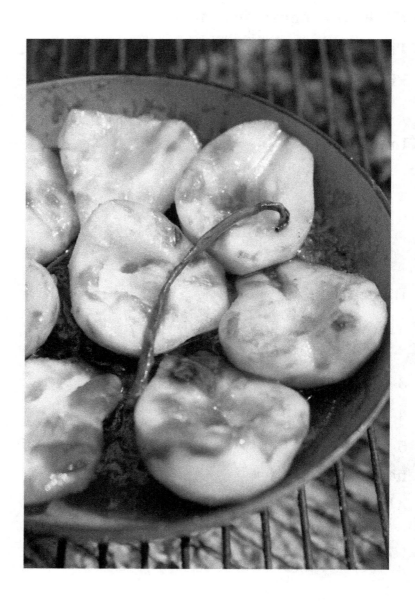

Cilantro And Avocado Platter

Time To Prepare: ten minutes

Time to Cook: 0 minutes

Yield: Servings 6

Ingredients:
- ¼ cup of fresh cilantro, chopped
- ½ a lime, juiced
- 1 big ripe tomato, chopped
- 1 green bell pepper, chopped
- 1 sweet onion, chopped
- 2 avocados, peeled, pitted and diced
- Salt and pepper as required

Directions:

1. Take a moderate-sized container and put in onion, bell pepper, tomato, avocados, lime and cilantro

2. Mix thoroughly and give it a toss

3. Sprinkle with salt and pepper in accordance with your taste

4. Serve and enjoy!

Cool Garbanzo and Spinach Beans

Time To Prepare: 5-ten minutes

Time to Cook: 0 minute

Yield: Servings 4

Ingredients:
- ½ onion, diced
- ½ teaspoon cumin
- 1 tablespoon olive oil
- 10 ounces spinach, chopped
- 12 ounces garbanzo beans

Directions:
1. Take a frying pan and put in olive oil

2. Put it on moderate to low heat

3. Put in onions, garbanzo and cook for five minutes

4. Mix in cumin, garbanzo beans, spinach and flavor with sunflower seeds

5. Use a spoon to smash gently

6. Cook meticulously

7. Serve and enjoy

Creamy Polenta

Time To Prepare: 8 minutes

Time to Cook: forty-five minutes

Yield: Servings: 4

Ingredients:

- ½ cup cream
- 1 ½ cup water
- 1 cup polenta
- 1/3 cup Parmesan, grated
- 2 cups chicken stock

Directions:

1. Put polenta in the pot.

2. Put in water, chicken stock, cream, and Parmesan.

3. Mix up polenta well.

4. Then preheat the oven to 355F.

5. Cook polenta in your oven for about forty-five minutes.

6. Mix up the cooked meal with the help of the spoon cautiously before you serve

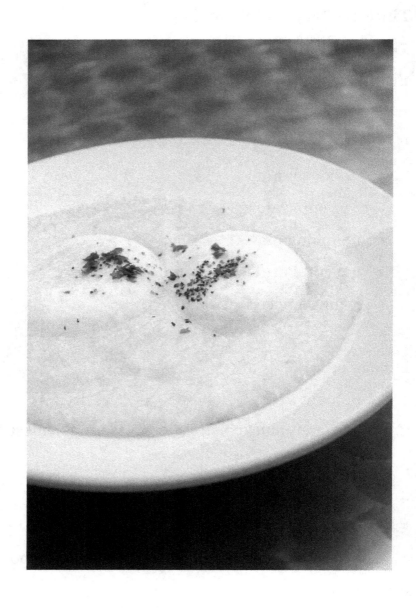

Cucumber Yogurt Salad with Mint

Time To Prepare: ten minutes

Time to Cook: 0 minutes

Yield: Servings 2

Ingredients:

- ¼ cup organic coconut milk
- ¼ cup organic mint leaves
- ¼ teaspoon pink Himalayan sea salt
- ½ cup chopped organic red onion
- 1 tablespoon extra virgin olive oil
- 1 tablespoon plain organic goat yogurt
- 1 teaspoon organic dill weed
- 2 chopped organic cucumbers
- 3 tablespoons fresh organic lime juice

Directions:

1. Cut the red onion, dill, cucumbers, and mint and mix them in a big container.

2. Blend them until they're smooth.

3. Top the dressing onto the cucumber salad and mix meticulously.

4. Chill for a minimum 1 hour and serve. Enjoy!

Farro Salad with Arugula

Time To Prepare: ten minutes

Time to Cook: thirty-five minutes

Yield: Servings 2

Ingredients:
- ½ cup farro
- ½ teaspoon ground black pepper
- ½ teaspoon Italian seasoning
- ½ teaspoon olive oil
- 1 ½ cup chicken stock
- 1 cucumber, chopped
- 1 tablespoon lemon juice
- 1 teaspoon salt
- 2 cups arugula, chopped

Directions:

1. Mix together farro, salt, and chicken stock and move mixture in the pan.

2. Close the lid and boil it for a little more than half an hour.

3. In the meantime, place all rest of the ingredients in the salad container.

4. Chill the farro to room temperature and put it in the salad container too.

5. Mix up the salad well.

Fresh Strawberry Salsa

Time To Prepare: ten minutes

Time to Cook: 0 minutes

Yield: Servings 6-8

Ingredients:
- ¼ cup fresh lime juice
- ½ cup fresh cilantro
- ½ cup red onion, finely chopped
- ½ teaspoon lime zest, grated
- 1-2 jalapeños, deseeded, finely chopped
- 2 kiwi fruit, peeled, chopped
- 2 pounds fresh ripe strawberries, hulled, chopped
- 2 teaspoons pure raw honey

Directions:

1. Put in lime juice, lime zest and honey into a big container and whisk well.

2. Put in remaining ingredients then mix thoroughly.

3. Cover and set aside for a while for the flavors to set in and serve

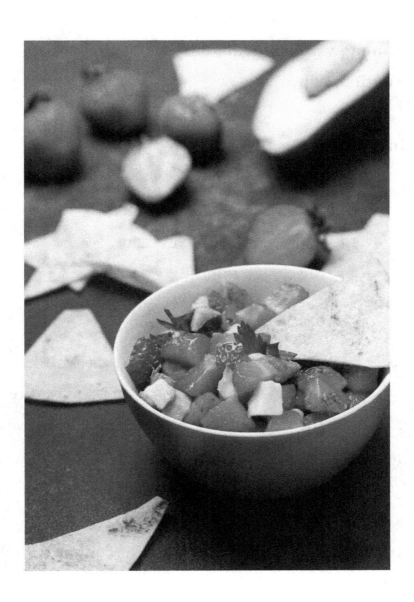

Green Beans

Time To Prepare: five minutes

Time to Cook: ten minutes

Yield: Servings 5

Ingredients:

- ½ teaspoon kosher salt
- ½ teaspoon of red pepper flakes
- 1½ lbs. green beans, trimmed
- 2 garlic cloves, minced
- 2 tablespoons of extra-virgin olive oil
- 2 tablespoons of water

Directions:

1. Heat oil in a frying pan on medium temperature.

2. Include the pepper flake. Stir to coat in the olive oil.

3. Include the green beans. Cook for seven minutes. Stir frequently.

4. The beans must be brown in some areas.

5. Put in the salt and garlic. Cook for a minute, while stirring.

6. Pour water and cover instantly. Cook covered for 1 more minute.

Hot Pink Coconut Slaw

Time To Prepare: five minutes

Time to Cook: 0 minutes

Yield: Servings 3

Ingredients:
- ¼ cup fresh cilantro, chopped
- ¼ teaspoon salt
- ½ cup big coconut flakes, unsweetened or shredded coconut, unsweetened
- ½ cup radish, thinly cut or shredded carrots
- ½ small jalapeño, deseeded, discard membranes, chopped
- ½ tablespoon honey or maple syrup
- 1 cup red onion, thinly cut
- 1 tablespoon olive oil
- 2 cups purple cabbage, thinly cut
- 2 tablespoons apple cider vinegar
- 2 tablespoons lime juice

Directions:
1. Combine all ingredients into a container and toss thoroughly.

2. Cover and set aside for about forty minutes.

3. Toss thoroughly before you serve.

Mascarpone Couscous

Time To Prepare: fifteen minutes

Time to Cook: 7.5 hours

Yield: Servings 4

Ingredients:

- ½ cup mascarpone
- 1 cup couscous
- 1 teaspoon ground paprika
- 1 teaspoon salt
- 3 ½ cup chicken stock

Directions:

1. Put chicken stock and mascarpone in the pan and bring the liquid to boil.

2. Put in salt and ground paprika. Stir gently and simmer for a minute.

3. Take off the liquid from the heat and put in couscous. Stir thoroughly and close the lid. Leave couscous for about ten minutes.

4. Mix the cooked side dish well before you serve.

Mushroom Millet

Time To Prepare:ten minutes

Time to Cook: fifteen minutes

Yield: Servings 3

Ingredients:
- ¼ cup mushrooms, cut
- ½ cup millet
- ¾ cup onion, diced
- 1 cup of water
- 1 tablespoon olive oil
- 1 teaspoon butter
- 1 teaspoon salt
- 3 tablespoons milk

Directions:
1. Pour olive oil in the frying pan then put the onion.

2. Put in mushrooms and roast the vegetables for about ten minutes over the moderate heat. Stir them occasionally.

3. In the meantime, pour water in the pan. Put in millet and salt.

4. Cook the millet with the closed lid for fifteen minutes over the moderate heat.

5. Then put in the cooked mushroom mixture in the millet. Put in milk and butter. Mix up the millet well.

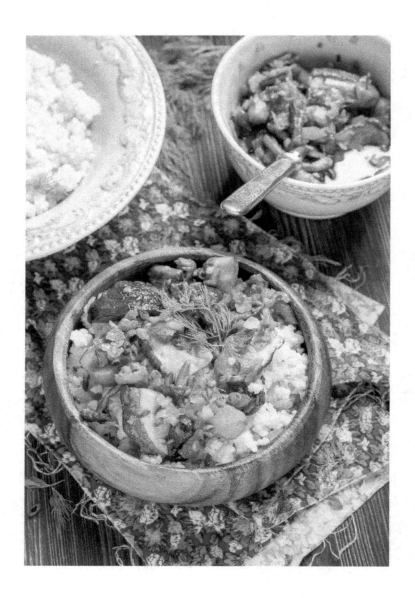

Parmesan Roasted Broccoli

Time To Prepare: ten minutes

Time to Cook: twenty minutes

Yield: Servings: 6

Ingredients:

- ½ teaspoon of Italian seasoning
- 1 tablespoon of lemon juice
- 1 tablespoon parsley, chopped
- 3 tablespoons of olive oil
- 3 tablespoons of vegan parmesan, grated
- 4 cups of broccoli florets
- Pepper and salt to taste

Directions:

1. Preheat the oven to 450 degrees F.

2. Apply cooking spray on your pan.

3. Keep the broccoli florets in a freezer bag. Now put in the Italian seasoning, olive oil, pepper, and salt. Seal your bag. Shake it. Coat well.

4. Pour your broccoli on the pan. It must be in a single layer. Bake for about twenty minutes. 5. Stir midway through. Take out from the oven.

6. Drizzle parsley and parmesan.

7. Sprinkle some lemon juice.

8. You can decorate with lemon wedges if you wish.

Red Cabbage with Cheese

Time To Prepare: five minutes

Time to Cook: twelve minutes

Yield: Servings 4

Ingredients:

- ¼ cup & 1 tbsp. of extra virgin olive oil
- ¼ tsp of freshly ground pepper
- ¼ tsp of salt
- 1 cup of walnuts
- 1 Tbsp. of crumbled blue cheese
- 1 tbsp. of Dijon mustard
- 1 tsp of butter
- 2 thinly cut scallions
- 3 tbsp. of pure maple syrup
- 3 tbsp. of red wine vinegar
- 8 cups of red cabbage, thinly cut

Directions:
For the vinaigrette:

1. Combine the blue cheese, ¼ cup of olive oil, mustard, vinegar, salt, and pepper in a food processor or blender until the mixture has a creamy consistency.

For the salad:

1. Put parchment paper near the stove.

2. Heat 1 tbsp. of oil on moderate heat in a moderate-sized frying pan and mix in the walnuts, cooking them for approximately 2 minutes.

3. Now mix salt and pepper, sprinkle maple syrup and cook for approximately three to five minutes while stirring the mixture up to the nuts are uniformly coated.

4. Move to the paper and pour the rest of the syrup over them using a spoon.

5. Separate the nuts and cool down for approximately five minutes.

6. In a big container, put in the cabbage and scallions and toss them with the vinaigrette.

7. Put in the walnuts and blue cheese as toppings.

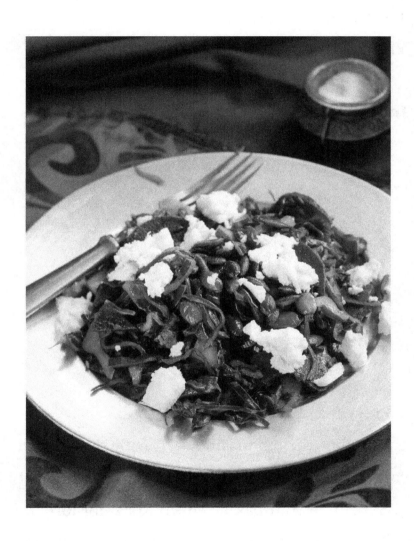

Roasted Carrots

Time To Prepare: ten minutes

Time to Cook: forty minutes

Yield: Servings 4

Ingredients:
- ¼ teaspoon ground pepper
- ½ teaspoon rosemary, chopped
- ½ teaspoon salt
- 1 onion, peeled & cut
- 1 teaspoon thyme, chopped
- 2 tablespoons of extra-virgin olive oil
- 8 carrots, peeled & cut

Directions:
1. Preheat the oven to 425 degrees F.

2. Combine the onions and carrots by tossing in a container with rosemary, thyme, pepper, and salt.

3. Spread on your baking sheet. Roast for forty minutes.

4. The onions and carrots must be browning and soft

Roasted Parsnips

Time To Prepare: five minutes

Time to Cook: thirty minutes

Yield: Servings 4

Ingredients:
- 1 tablespoon of extra-virgin olive oil
- 1 teaspoon of kosher salt
- 1½ teaspoon of Italian seasoning
- 2 lbs. parsnips Chopped parsley for decoration

Directions:
1. Preheat the oven to 400 degrees F.

2. Peel the parsnips. Cut them into one-inch chunks.

3. Now toss with the seasoning, salt, and oil in a container.

4. Spread this on your baking sheet. It must be in a single layer.

5. Roast for half an hour. Stir every ten minutes.

6. Move to a plate.

7. Decorate using parsley.

Shoepeg Corn Salad

Time To Prepare: ten minutes

Time to Cook: 0 minute

Yield: Servings 4

Ingredients:
- ¼ cup Greek yogurt
- ½ cup cherry tomatoes halved
- 1 cup shoepeg corn, drained
- 1 jalapeno pepper, chopped
- 1 tablespoon chives, chopped
- 1 tablespoon lemon juice
- 3 tablespoons fresh cilantro, chopped

Directions:
1. In the salad container, mix up together shoepeg corn, cherry tomatoes, jalapeno pepper, chives, and fresh cilantro.
2. Put in lemon juice and Greek yogurt.
3. Mix your salad well.
4. Put in your fridge and store it for maximum 1 day.

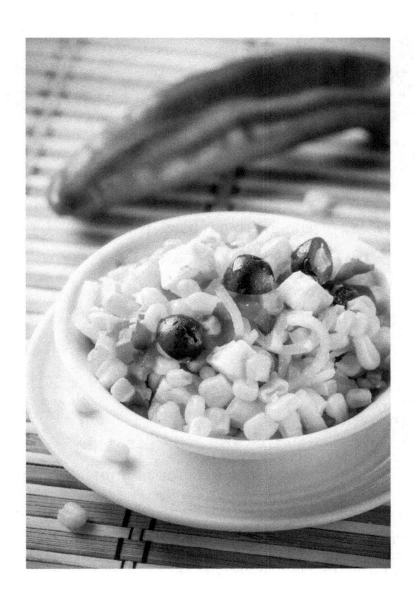

Spicy Barley

Time To Prepare: seven minutes

Time to Cook: 42 minutes

Yield: Servings 5

Ingredients:
- ½ teaspoon cayenne pepper
- ½ teaspoon chili pepper
- ½ teaspoon ground black pepper
- 1 cup barley
- 1 teaspoon butter
- 1 teaspoon olive oil
- 1 teaspoon salt
- 3 cups chicken stock

Directions:

1. Put barley and olive oil in the pan.

2. Roast barley on high heat for a minute. Stir it well.

3. Then put in salt, chili pepper, ground black pepper, cayenne pepper, and butter.

4. Put in chicken stock.

5. Close the lid and cook barley for forty minutes over the medium-low heat.

Spicy Wasabi Mayonnaise

Time To Prepare: fifteen minutes

Time to Cook: 0 minute

Yield: Servings 4

Ingredients:
- ½ tablespoon wasabi paste
- 1 cup mayonnaise

Directions:

1. Take a container and mix wasabi paste and

mayonnaise. Mix thoroughly

2. Allow it to chill, use as required

3. Serve and enjoy

Stir-Fried Farros

Time To Prepare: five minutes

Time to Cook: thirty-five minutes

Yield: Servings 2

Ingredients:
- ½ cup farro
- ½ teaspoon ground coriander
- ½ teaspoon paprika
- ½ teaspoon turmeric
- 1 ½ cup water
- 1 carrot, grated
- 1 tablespoon butter
- 1 teaspoon chili flakes
- 1 teaspoon salt
- 1 yellow onion, cut

Directions:
1. Put farro in the pan.

2. Put in water and salt.

3. Close the lid and boil it for half an hour In the meantime, toss the butter in the frying pan. 4. Heat it and put in cut onion and grated carrot.

5. Fry the vegetables for about ten minutes over the moderate heat.

6. Stir them with the help of spatula occasionally.

7. When the farro is cooked, put it in the roasted vegetables and mix up well.

8. Cook stir-fried farro for five minutes over the moderate to high heat.

Thyme with Honey-Roasted Carrots

Time To Prepare: five minutes

Time to Cook: thirty minutes

Yield: Servings 4

Ingredients:

- ½ teaspoon of sea salt
- ½ teaspoon thyme, dried
- 1 tablespoon of honey
- 1/5 lb. carrots, with the tops
- 2 tablespoons of olive oil

Directions:

1. Preheat the oven to 425 degrees F.

2. Place parchment paper on your baking sheet.

3. Toss your carrots with honey, oil, thyme, and salt. Coat well. Keep in a single layer.

4. Bake in the oven for half an hour

5. Allow to cool before you serve

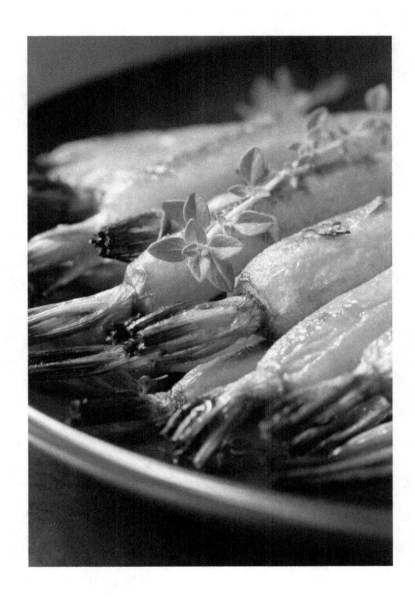

Wheatberry Salad

Time To Prepare: ten minutes

Time to Cook: 50 minutes

Yield: Servings 2

Ingredients:

- ¼ cup fresh parsley, chopped
- ¼ cup of wheat berries
- 1 cup of water
- 1 tablespoon canola oil
- 1 tablespoon chives, chopped
- 1 teaspoon chili flakes
- 1 teaspoon salt
- 2 oz. pomegranate seeds
- 2 tablespoons walnuts, chopped

Directions:

1. Put wheat berries and water in the pan.

2. Put in salt and simmer the ingredients for about fifty minutes over the moderate heat. In the meantime, mix up together walnuts, chives, parsley, pomegranate seeds, and chili flakes.

3. When the wheatberry is cooked, move it in the walnut mixture.

4. Put in canola oil and mix up the salad well.

Balsamic Vinaigrette

Time To Prepare: ten minutes

Time to Cook: 0 minutes

Yield: Servings 2-4

Ingredients:

- ¼ tsp of freshly ground black pepper
- ½ cup of extra-virgin olive oil
- ½ cup of rice vinegar
- 1 clove of freshly minced garlic
- 1 tbsp. of honey or maple syrup
- 1 tsp of sea or kosher salt
- 2 tsp of Dijon mustard

Directions:

1. Put all ingredients in a mason jar and cover firmly.

2. Shake thoroughly until all ingredients are blended.

3. Keep in your fridge for minimum 30 minutes before you serve to keep its freshness.

4. Serve with a salad or as your meat marinate.

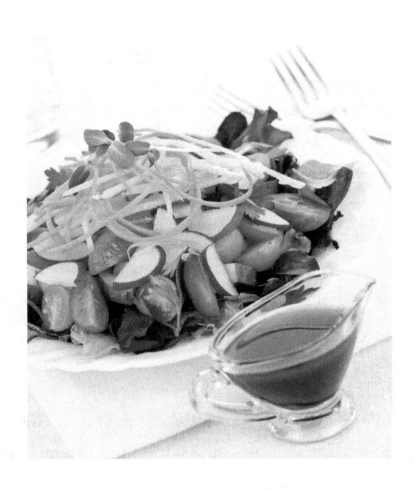

Cashew Ginger Dip

Time To Prepare: five minutes

Time to Cook: 0 minutes

Yield: Servings 1

Ingredients:

- ¼ cup filtered water

- ¼ teaspoon salt

- ½ teaspoon ground ginger

- 1 cup cashews, soaked in water for about twenty minutes and drained

- 1 tablespoon extra-virgin olive oil

- 1 teaspoon lemon juice

- 2 garlic cloves

- 2 teaspoons coconut aminos

- Pinch cayenne pepper

Directions:

1. In a blender or food processor, put together the cashews, garlic, water, olive oil, aminos, lemon juice, ginger, salt, and cayenne pepper.

2. Put in the mix in a container.

3. Cover and place in your fridge until chilled.

4. You can store it for 4-5 days in your fridge.

Creamy Homemade Greek Dressing

Time To Prepare: ten minutes

Time to Cook: 0 minutes

Yield: Servings 2-4

Ingredients:

- ¼ cup non-dairy milk (e.g., almond, rice milk)
- ½ cup of high-quality mayonnaise, without preservatives
- ½ tsp dried basil
- ½ tsp dried oregano
- ½ tsp parsley
- ½ tsp thyme
- 1/3 cup of extra-virgin olive oil
- 1/4 cup of white wine vinegar
- 2 cloves of garlic, minced
- 2 tbsp. of lemon or lime juice
- 2 tsp of honey
- A few tablespoons of water
- Some Kosher salt and pepper

Directions:

1. Put all together ingredients in a mason jar and shake, cover firmly, and shake thoroughly.

2. Place in your fridge for a few hours before you serve or serve instantly on your favorite vegetable or fruit salad.

3. Shake well before use.

4. Put it in your fridge for a maximum 5 days.

5. You may put in a few tablespoons of water to tune the consistency as per your preference.

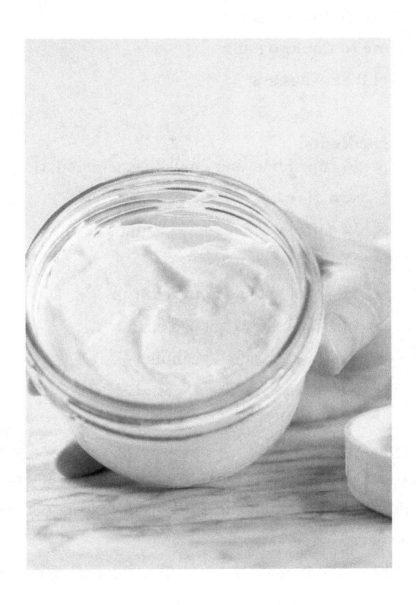

Creamy Siamese Dressing

Time To Prepare: ten minutes

Time to Cook: 0 minutes

Yield: Servings 2-4

Ingredients:
- ¼ cup of non-dairy milk (e.g., almond, rice, soymilk)
- ¼ cup of unsweetened peanut sauce
- 1 cup of mayonnaise
- 1 tbsp. of honey or maple syrup
- 1 tbsps. freshly chopped cilantro
- 2 tbsp. of unsalted peanuts
- 2 tbsp. rice vinegar

Directions:

1. Put all ingredients apart from the cilantro and peanuts into a blender and blend until the desired smoothness is achieved and creamy.

2. Next, put in the cilantro and peanuts and pulse the blender a few times until completely crushed and well blended.

3. Put in a mason jar and bring it in your fridge.

4. Serve with a garden salad, pasta or as a dipping sauce.

Dairy-Free Creamy Turmeric Dressing

Time To Prepare: ten minutes

Time to Cook: 0 minutes

Yield: Servings 2-4

Ingredients:

- ½ cup of extra-virgin olive oil
- ½ cup of tahini
- 1 tbsp. of turmeric powder
- 2 tbsp. of lemon juice
- 2 tsp of honey
- Some sea salt and pepper

Directions:

1. In a container, whisk all ingredients until well blended.

2. Store in a mason jar and place in your fridge for maximum 5 days.

Homemade Ginger Dressing

Time To Prepare: ten minutes

Time to Cook: 0 minutes

Yield: Servings 2-4

Ingredients:

- ¼ cup of chopped celery
- ¼ cup of honey or maple syrup
- ¼ cup of water
- ½ cup of chopped carrots
- ½ tsp of white pepper
- 1 cup of chopped onion
- 1 cup of extra-virgin olive oil
- 1 tsp of freshly minced garlic
- 1 tsp of kosher salt
- 2 ½ tbsp. of unsalted, gluten-free soy sauce
- 2 tbsp. of ketchup
- 2/3 cup of rice vinegar
- 6 tbsp. of freshly grated ginger

Directions:

1. Put the onion, ginger, celery, carrots, and garlic into a blender.

2. Blend until the mixture is fine but still lumpy from the small vegetable chunks.

3. Put in the vinegar, water, ketchup, soy sauce, honey or maple syrup, lemon juice, salt, and pepper.

4. Pulse until the ingredients are well blended.

5. Slowly put in the oil while blending, until everything is thoroughly combined.

6. The mixture must be runny but still grainy.

7. Serve with a winter salad.

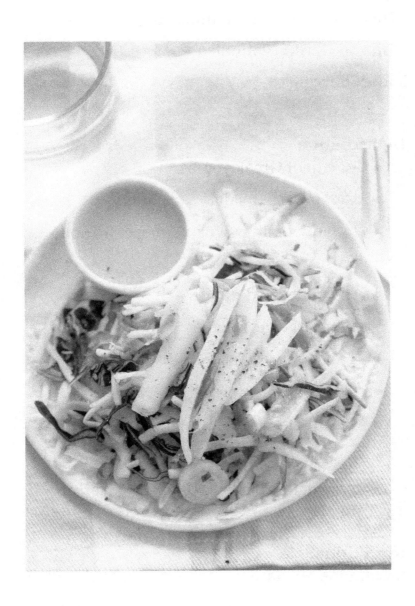

Homemade Ranch

Time To Prepare: ten minutes

Time to Cook: 0 minutes

Yield: Servings 2-4

Ingredients:
- ¼ cup of Greek yogurt
- ¼ tsp Kosher salt
- ½ cup of natural mayonnaise, without preservatives
- ½ tsp of dried dill
- ½ tsp of dried parsley
- ½ tsp of garlic powder
- ½ tsp of onion powder
- ¾ cup of non-dairy milk
- 1/8 tsp Freshly ground black pepper
- 2 tsp of dried chives

Directions:
1. Combine all ingredients apart from the milk into a medium container.
2. Mix together until well blended.

3. Put in the milk and mix thoroughly.

4. Pour in a mason jar or an airtight container.

5. Serve instantly or place in your fridge for maximum 2 hours to keep the freshness.

6. Put in your refrigerator for a maximum of 5 days.

7. Serve with a garden or fruit salad.

Soy with Honey and Ginger Glaze

Time To Prepare: ten minutes

Time to Cook: 0 minutes

Yield: Servings 2-4

Ingredients:
- ¼ cup of honey
- 1 tbsp. of rice vinegar
- 1 tsp of freshly grated ginger
- 2 tbsp. gluten-free soy sauce

Directions:

1. Put all together the ingredients into a small container and whisk well.

2. Serve with vegetables, chickens, or seafood.

3. Keep the glaze in a mason jar, firmly covered, and place in your fridge for maximum four days.

Tahini Dip

Time To Prepare: ten minutes

Time to Cook: 0 minutes

Yield: Servings 2-4

Ingredients:
- ¼ cup of tahini
- ½ tsp of maple syrup
- 1 small grated or thoroughly minced clove of garlic (this is optional)
- 1 tbsp. of apple cider vinegar
- 1 tbsp. of freshly squeezed lemon juice
- 1 tbsp. of tamari
- 1 tsp of finely grated ginger, or ½ tsp of ground ginger
- 1 tsp of turmeric
- 1/3 cup of water

Directions:
1. Blend or whisk all ingredients together.

2. Place the dressing in an airtight container then place in your fridge for approximately 5 days. Enjoy!

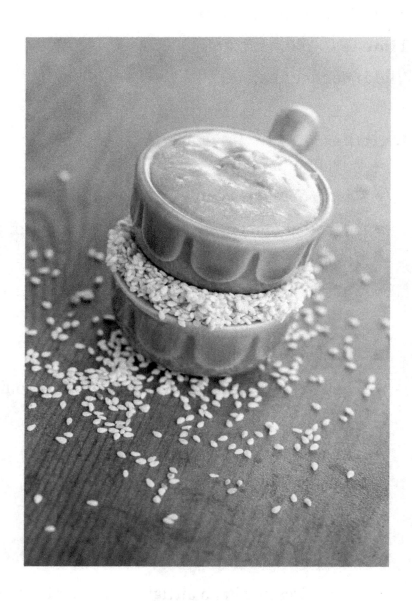

SNACKS

Almond and Honey Homemade Bar

Time To Prepare: fifteen minutes + thirty minutes refrigerator time

Time to Cook: fifteen minutes

Yield: Servings 8

Ingredients:
- ¼ cup almond butter
- ¼ cup honey
- ¼ cup sugar (or another sweetener to your taste in adjusted amount)
- ¼ cup sunflower seeds
- ½ teaspoon vanilla extract
- 1 cup oats
- 1 cup whole-grain puffed cereal (unsweetened)
- 1 tbsp. flaxseeds
- 1 tbsp. sesame seeds
- 1/3 cup apricots (dried and chopped)
- 1/3 cup currants
- 1/3 cup raisins (chopped)

- 1/8 tsp salt
- A ¼ cup of almonds

Directions:

1. Preheat your oven to 350 degrees Fahrenheit.

2. Place a baking paper on an 8-inch pan or coat it with cooking spray/oil.

3. Combine the almonds, oats, and seeds and spread the mixture on a rimmed baking sheet.

4. Bake the mixture until you notice that the oats are mildly toasted (for approximately ten minutes).

5. Move the mixture to a container. Put in cereal, raisins, currants, and apricots to the container. Toss thoroughly to blend.

6. Mix honey, almond butter, vanilla, salt, and sugar in a deep cooking pan.

7. Heat on moderate heat. Stir regularly for 2-5 minutes until you see light bubbles.

8. Once you notice the bubbles, pour the mixture over the dry mixture with apricots and oats you prepared previously.

9. Mix thoroughly using a spatula. There mustn't be any dry spots.

10. Move the new mixture to the previously prepared pan.

11. Push it to the pan to make a firm and flat layer.

12. Place in your refrigerator for half an hour. Chop the layer into eight equal bars or squares, to your taste.

13. Consume instantly or place in your refrigerator up to seven days

Anti-Inflammatory Key Lime Pie

Time To Prepare: twenty minutes + thirty-five minutes refrigerator time

Time to Cook: 0 Yield: Servings 8

Ingredients:

- ½ cup honey
- ½ cup Medjool dates, chopped and pitted
- 1 cup unsweetened shredded coconut
- 1 cup walnuts
- 1 teaspoon lime zest
- 1/4 teaspoon sea salt
- 3 firm avocados
- 3 tablespoons lime juice
- Lime slices
- Pinch of sea salt

Directions:

1. Use a food processor to put all together the walnuts, coconut, and the salt, then pulse until crudely ground.

2. Place the dates and pulse until the mixture resembles bread crumbs, trying to stick together.

3. Push the mixture into the edges and bottom of a non-stick greased 9-inch pie pan.

4. Use your fingers or the back of a spoon to press the crust into a uniform layer.

5. Bring the crust into the freezer for minimum fifteen minutes while preparing the filling.

6. Use the food processor again and mix the avocado, honey, lime juice, lime zest, and salt.

7. Process until the desired smoothness is achieved.

8. Pour the filling into the now-chilled pie crust and place it in your fridge for about twenty minutes.

9. Decorate using fresh lime slices and serve cold.

11. Store any leftovers in your fridge

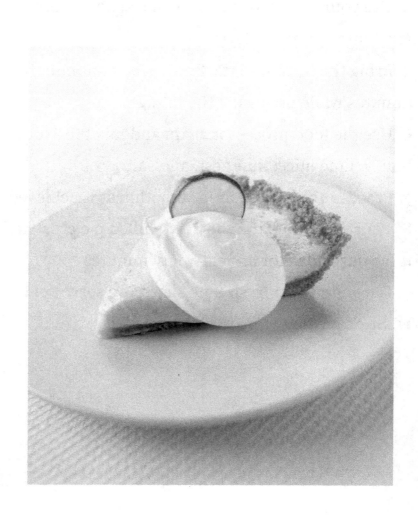

Apple Crisp

Time To Prepare: fifteen minutes

Time to Cook: twenty-five minutes

Yield: Servings 6-8

Ingredients:
Topping:

- 1 ½ cups old-fashioned rolled oats

- 1 teaspoon salt ½ cup stevia

- 2 teaspoons ground cinnamon

- 1 cup nuts, crudely chopped

- 3 tablespoon melted coconut oil.

- 1/3 cup almond meal

- 2/3 cup shredded, unsweetened coconut

- 1/4 teaspoon ground nutmeg

Apple filling:

- ½ cup stevia

- 1 tablespoon ground cinnamon

- 1 teaspoon vanilla

- 1/4 cup arrowroot flour

- 1/4 teaspoon salt

- 10 tart apples

- 2 tablespoons fresh-squeezed lemon juice

- 3 tablespoons melted coconut oil

- The zest of 1 orange

Directions:

1. Set the oven to 350 F then grease a 9 by a 13-inch baking pan with coconut oil.

2. Put together the topping ingredients in a container, then mix and save for later.

3. Combine the filling ingredients (except for the apples) in a second big container.

4. Leave the skins on the apples, if you wish. Core them and slice super slim (1/8 inch thick).

5. Toss the apples in the filling ingredients to coat uniformly.

6. Put the apple mixture in a baking pan and spread the topping over it all, pushing down tightly.

7. Put in your oven with a pan underneath to catch any drips.

8. Bake for about twenty-five minutes or until the topping is brown and juices are bubbling.

Apples must be tender. Cool slightly on a rack then serve

Avocado and Egg Sandwich

Time To Prepare: ten minutes

Time to Cook: 0 minutes

Yield: Servings 2

Ingredients:

- ½ lime juice
- 1 avocado (ripe)
- 1 egg, organic
- 1 scallion
- 2 radishes
- 2 slices of whole wheat, seed bread
- A pinch of salt (sea or Himalayan)
- Black pepper – to your taste
- Mixed seeds – to your choice

Directions:

1. Peel the avocado.

2. Boil the egg (soft boiled).

3. Chop the radishes to thin slices.

4. Dice the scallion (finely).

5. Mix avocado, salt, and lime juice in a container.

6. Mash the mixture meticulously.

7. Spread the mixture onto the bread.

8. Put in some radish.

9. Put tender boiled eggs on top.

10. Put in some scallion, seeds, and pepper.

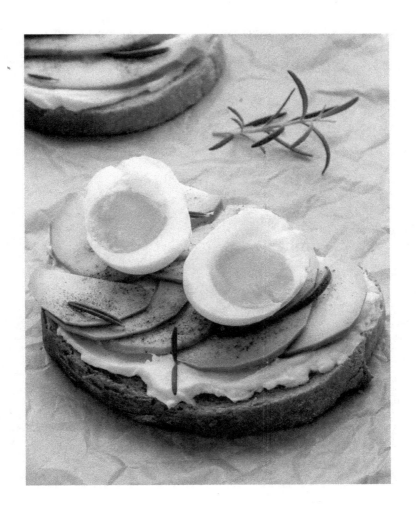

Avocado with Tomatoes and Cucumber

Time To Prepare: ten minutes

Time to Cook: 0 minutes

Yield: Servings 2

Ingredients:
- ¼ cup cilantro
- ¼ cup olives – to your choice
- ½ red onion
- 1 cucumber
- 1 lemon
- 1 Tbsp. turmeric
- 1/8 cup parsley
- 2 avocados
- 4 Roma tomatoes
- Salt and pepper – to your taste

Directions:
1. Dice the tomatoes, cucumber, avocado, and olives.

2. Cut the cilantro, parsley, and onion.

3. Put in the above ingredients into a container.

4. Squeeze the lemon juice then put it into the vegetables.

5. Put in olive oil, turmeric, salt, and pepper. Toss thoroughly.

6. Consume instantly after putting in lemon juice and olive oil.

If you prefer to consume the salad later, put in the dressing instantly before consuming it.

Berry Delight

Time To Prepare: fifteen minutes

Time to Cook: 0 minutes

Yield: Servings 6

Ingredients:

- ¼ cup of raw honey
- 1 cup of fresh organic blackberries
- 1 cup of fresh organic blueberries
- 1 cup of fresh organic raspberries
- 1 tablespoon of cinnamon

Directions:

1. Mix all the berries together in a big container, put in the honey, and slowly stir.

2. Drizzle with the cinnamon.

Blueberry & Chia Flax Seed Pudding

Time To Prepare: ten minutes

Time to Cook: fifteen minutes

Yield: Servings 4

Ingredients:

- ¼ cup of blueberries
- 2 cups of almond milk
- 3 tablespoons of chia seeds
- 3 tablespoons of ground flaxseed

Directions:

1. Warm a pan on moderate heat then put all together of the ingredients apart from the blueberries.

2. Stir all the ingredients until the pudding is thick, this will take around three minutes.

Place the pudding into a container then top with blueberries.

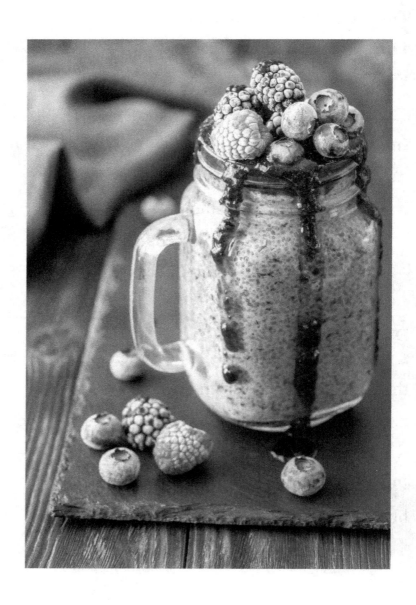

Brownies Avocado

Time To Prepare: ten minutes

Time to Cook: twenty-five minutes

Yield: Servings 6-8

Ingredients:

- ½ cup almond meal
- 1 ½ teaspoon instant coffee (with or without caffeine, as you wish)
- 2 teaspoons ground cinnamon
- ½ teaspoon salt 2 cups nuts or seeds, chopped
- 1 avocado
- 1 apple, cored and chopped, with the skin on
- 1 cup cooked and diced sweet potato
- 4 tablespoons ground chia seeds
- 1 teaspoon vanilla
- ½ cup almond butter
- ½ cup coconut butter, softened
- 1/4 cup coconut oil
- 2 1/4 cup stevia
- 3/4 cup cocoa powder

Directions:

1. Set the oven to 350F then line a 9 by 13-inch pan with parchment.

2. Allow it to overlap the sides to make handles for lifting the brownies out when done.

3. In a container, mix the almond meal, cocoa, coffee, cinnamon, salt, and nuts. Whisk and save for later.

4. Bring the remaining ingredients in a food processor and mix until the desired smoothness is achieved.

5. Put in the ingredients in the container and pulse. This combination must be lumpy.

6. Pour into the pan and bake for minimum twenty-five minutes.

7. Allow to cool and chill in your fridge for a couple of hours before cutting.

8. The baked product will be a little gooey, so refrigerating it makes the brownies easier to cut. The chilled results will be fairly crumbly.

Brussels Sprout Chips

Time To Prepare: ten minutes

Time to Cook: ten minutes

Yield: Servings 4

Ingredients:
- 2 cups Brussels sprout leaves
- 2 tablespoons ghee
- Kosher salt
- Lemon zest

Directions:
1. Set the oven to 350F, then cover two cookie sheets using parchment paper.
2. Place the leaves in a huge container and pour melted ghee over the top, and put in salt.
3. Bake for minimum 8 to ten minutes or until the leaves are crunchy. If they are tender at all, put them back in your oven.
4. While still hot, drizzle the lemon zest over the leaves.
5. Serve warm

Candied Dates

Time To Prepare: five minutes

Time to Cook: 0 minutes

Yield: Servings 2

Ingredients:

- 2 tablespoons of dark cocoa nibs
- 2 tablespoons of peanut butter
- 4 pitted Medjool dates

Directions:

1. Cut the pitted dates in half, and spread half a tablespoon of peanut butter on each date.

2. Top each date with half a tablespoon of dark cocoa nibs.

3. Split the candied dates between two plates, and enjoy!

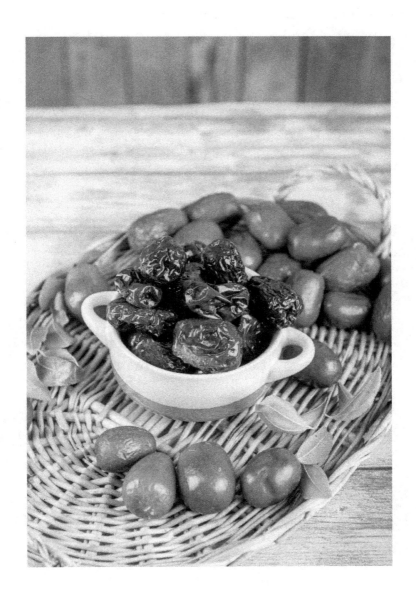

Cashew "Humus"

Time To Prepare: ten minutes

Time to Cook: 0 minutes

Yield: Servings 1

Ingredients:

- ¼ Cup Water
- ¼ Teaspoon Sea Salt, Fine
- ½ Teaspoon Ground Ginger
- 1 Cup Cashews, Raw & Soaked in Water for fifteen Minutes & Drained
- 1 Tablespoon Olive Oil
- 1 Teaspoon Lemon juice, Fresh
- 2 Cloves Garlic
- 2 Teaspoon Coconut Aminos
- Pinch Cayenne Pepper

Directions:

1. Blend all ingredients together, and ensure to scrape the sides.

2. Continue to combine until the desired smoothness is achieved, and then place in your fridge it before you serve

Cauliflower Snacks

Time To Prepare: ten minutes

Time to Cook: 60 minutes

Yield: Servings 4

Ingredients:
- 1 head of cauliflower
- 1 teaspoon salt
- 4 tablespoons extra virgin olive oil

Directions:
1. Set the oven to 425F, then prepare two cookie sheets by lining them using parchment paper.
2. Trim off the cauliflower florets and discard the core.
3. Chop the florets into golf-ball-sized pieces.
4. Put the cauliflower in a container, and pour olive oil over them and drizzle with salt. Mix to coat.
5. Spread in a single layer, not touching.
6. Roast approximately 1 hour flipping the cauliflower three to four times until a golden-brown color is achieved.
7. Serve warm

Chewy Blackberry Leather

Time To Prepare: fifteen minutes

Time to Cook: 5-6 hours

Yield: Servings 8

Ingredients:
- ¼ cup of raw honey
- 1 tbsp. of fresh mint leaves
- 1 tsp. of ground cinnamon
- 1/8 tsp. of fresh lemon juice
- 2 cups of fresh blackberries

Directions:
1. Set the oven to 170F. Coat a baking sheet using parchment paper.
2. Use a food processor to put all ingredients and pulse till smooth.
3. Take the mixture onto the readied baking sheet and, using the backside of a spoon, smooth the top.
4. Bake for approximately 5-6 hours.
5. Chop the leather into equal-sized strips.
6. Now, roll each rectangle to make fruit rolls

Coco Cherry Bake-less Bars

Time To Prepare: ten minutes

Time to Cook: 0 minutes

Yield: Servings 6

Ingredients:

- ¼-cup pure maple syrup

- ⅓ -cup coconut, unsweetened and shredded

- ⅓ -cup dried cherries or cranberries

- ⅓ -cup ground flaxseed

- ½-cup almond butter

- 1- cup old-fashioned oats

- 1-Tbsp almond milk

- 1-Tbsp vanilla extract

- 3-scoops vanilla plant-based Protein powder

Directions:

1. Coat a loaf pan using parchment paper.

2. Mix in the first four ingredients in your blender.

3. Blend until the mixture becomes powdery.

4. Move the mixture to a mixing container.

5. Put in all the rest of the ingredients.

6. Mix thoroughly until meticulously blended.

7. Put the mixture in the pan, and press down onto a consistently flat surface.

8. Freeze for thirty minutes before cutting into six bars.

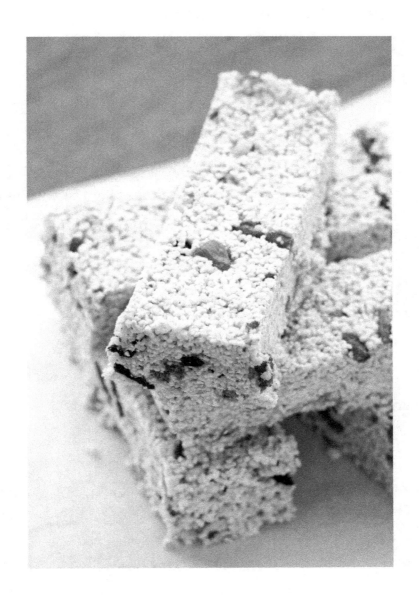

Cottage Cheese with Apple Sauce

Time To Prepare: five minutes

Time to Cook: 0 minutes

Yield: Servings 2

Ingredients:

- ½ teaspoon cinnamon powder
- 5-6 tablespoons cottage cheese two to three tablespoons applesauce or more if required

Directions:

1. Split the cottage cheese into 2 bowls.

2. Spread applesauce over the cottage cheese.

3. Drizzle ¼ teaspoon cinnamon powder on each before you serve.

Cucumber Yogurt

Time To Prepare: five minutes

Time to Cook: 0 minutes

Yield: Servings 1

Ingredients:

- 1 cup cucumbers, skin removed and chopped in chunks
- 1 teaspoon fresh dill, chopped fine
- 1/4 cup fat-free Greek yogurt
- 2 tablespoons chopped cashews
- 2 teaspoons fresh-squeezed lemon juice

Directions:

1. Peel and cut the cucumbers, then put them in a container.

2. Put in the cashews, yogurt, lemon juice, and dill.

3. Mix thoroughly, grab a spoon, and enjoy.

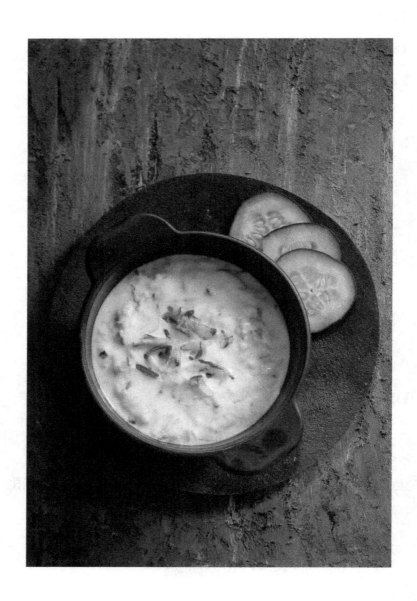

Dried Dates & Turmeric Truffles

Time To Prepare: fifteen minutes

Time to Cook: 0 minutes

Yield: Servings 4

Ingredients:

- ¼-tsp black pepper
- ⅓ -cup walnuts
- ½-cup rolled oats
- ¾-cup dates, pitted
- 1- Tbsp turmeric powder + more for rolling

Directions:

1. Mix in all the ingredients, excluding the dates in a food processor.

2. Blend until meticulously blended.

3. Put in the dates progressively until forming into the dough.

4. Shape and roll balls from the mixture.

5. Roll each ball with the additional turmeric powder until coating fully.

6. Store the truffles in an airtight jar until ready to serve.

Grams Easy Peasy Ginger Date

Time To Prepare: twenty minutes

Time to Cook: ten minutes

Yield: Servings 8

Ingredients:
- ¼ cup Almond milk
- ¾ cup Dates
- 1 or 1 ½ cup Almonds or almond flour
- 1 tsp. Ground ginger

Directions:
1. Preheat your oven to 350°F.

2. If you're using fresh almonds, put it through a blender to turn it to almond flour.

3. Blitz for a couple of minutes or so until it looks and feels smooth.

4. Do not blitz for too long, or you might end up making nut butter.

5. Now that you have your almond powder put it in a container and set it aside.

6. Pour the dates and almond milk into your blender and pulse for five minutes.

7. If it doesn't resemble a paste, pulse for another two minutes.

8. Pour in the ground ginger and almond flour.

9. Pulse for three to four minutes to combine.

10. Place the mixture in a baking dish and bake for approximately twenty minutes.

11. Take out of the oven and leave to cool before cutting into bits.

12. Serve or store.

Energy Dates Balls

Time To Prepare: ten minutes

Time to Cook: twenty-five minutes

Yield: Servings 7

Ingredients:
- ¼ cup of fresh lemon juice
- ½ cup of shredded sweetened coconut
- 1 cup of pitted and chopped dates
- 1 cup of toasted almonds

Directions:
1. Coat a big baking sheet using a parchment paper. Keep aside.

2. Use a food processor to add almonds and pulse till chopped crudely.

3. Put in dates and lemon juice and pulse till a tender dough forms.

4. Make equal sized balls from the mixture. In a shallow, dish place shredded coconut.

5. Roll the balls in shredded coconut uniformly.

6. Place the balls onto the baking sheet in a single layer.

7. Place in your fridge to set completely before you serve.

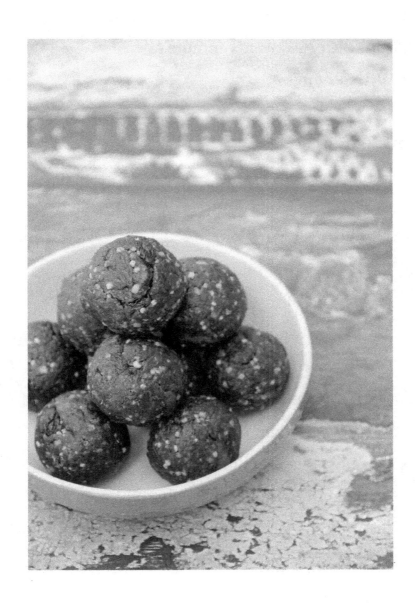

Flourless & Flaky Muffin Munchies

Time To Prepare: twenty-five minutes

Time to Cook: twenty minutes

Yield: Servings 4

Ingredients:

- ⅛-tsp baking soda
- ¼-cup peanut butter or allergy-friendly substitution
- ¼-cup pure maple syrup or honey
- ¼-tsp salt
- ½-cup quick oats or quinoa flakes, loosely packed
- ¾-tsp baking powder
- 1-cup white beans, cooked
- 1-pc medium mashed banana, very ripe
- 2-tsp pure vanilla extract
- A handful of mini chocolate chips, crushed walnuts, shredded coconut, pinch cinnamon, etc. (not necessary)

Directions:
1. Preheat your oven to 350 F.

2. Coat 8-muffin cups with glassine.

3. Mix all the ingredients in your blender.

4. Blend to a smooth consistency.

5. Pour the mixture into the muffin cups at ⅔ full.

6. Place the cups in your oven, and bake for about twenty minutes.

7. Allow the muffins to sit and cool for about twenty minutes.

Ginger Turmeric Protein: Bars

Time To Prepare: ten minutes + 20 cooling time

Time to Cook: twenty-five minutes

Yield: Servings 7

Ingredients:
- ½ cup coconut
- 1 cup cashews
- 1 scoop turmeric Protein bone broth
- 1 Tbsp. ginger
- 1/3 cup sunflower butter
- 2 Tbsp. maple syrup

Directions:

1. Put in coconut pieces and cashews to a blender or food processor.

2. Use the pulse option to obtain a coarse mixture.

3. Put in butter, broth, maple syrup, and ginger and pulse the mixture to make a coarse, yet even and fairly sticky mass.

4. Evenly put the mixture into a baking pan (8x8 inches) with your hands or a spoon.

5. Push tightly to the baking pan.

6. Bring it in a fridge and allow it to cool for about twenty minutes.

7. Chop the mixture into even squares.

8. You can consume instantly or store in a glass container in the refrigerator (up to 7 days

Hummus with Celery

Time To Prepare: fifteen minutes

Time to Cook: 0 minutes

Yield: Servings 4

Ingredients:

- 3 cloves of garlic, crushed
- 2 tablespoons extra virgin olive oil
- ½ teaspoon salt
- ½ teaspoon cumin
- 1 (fifteen–ounce) can chickpeas
- two to three tablespoons water
- Dash of paprika 6 stalks celery, cut into two-inch pieces
- 3 tablespoons salsa
- 1/4 cup lemon juice
- 1/4 cup tahini

Directions:

1. Using a food processor mix the lemon juice and tahini for approximately one minute, until it is smooth.

2. Scrape the sides down and process for 30 more seconds.

3. Put in the garlic, olive oil, salt, and cumin. Blend for approximately one minute.

4. Drain the chickpeas, put the half of them on the food processor, and blend for one more minute.

5. Scrape down the sides, put in the other half of the chickpeas, and pulse until smooth, approximately 2 minutes.

6. If it's a little too thick, put in water, 1 tablespoon at a time until you reach the desired consistency.

7. Fill the celery sticks with hummus and drizzle paprika on top.

8. Serve with salsa for dipping.

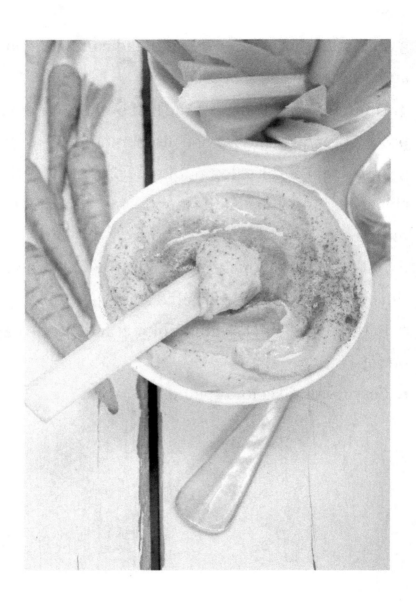

Notes